# Cancer and Nutrition

# Cancer and Nutrition

Elizabeth Somer, MA, RD

Publisher: Robert H. Garrison, Jr., MA, RPh
Editor In Chief: Elizabeth Somer, MA, RD
Managing Editor: Lisa M. Moye
Editorial Director: Janet L. Haley
Art Director: Scott Mayeda
Production Directors: Jeff Elkind, Irene Villa
Copy Editors: Norma Trost Foor, Jean Forsythe, Mary Houser,
               Stephen C. Schneider, R. H. Garrison, Sr., RPh
Cover Design: Stefanko & Hetz, Jeff Elkind
Photography: Bob and Irene Nishihira, Carlsbad, CA
Illustration: Walter Stuart

Copyright © 1986 by Health Media of America, Inc.

For information regarding volume purchase discounts contact:
    Health Media of America, Inc.
    11300 Sorrento Valley Road, Suite 250
    San Diego, CA 92121

Printed in the United States of America.

ISBN 0-937325-05-8

# Contents

## Introduction

**Section I:**
**What Is Cancer?** . . . . . . . . . . . . . . . . . . . . . . . . . . . . 1

**Section II:**
**Nutrition and the Prevention of Cancer** . . . . . . . . 7
    Ideal Body Weight . . . . . . . . . . . . . . . . . . . . . . 7
    Dietary Fat and Cholesterol . . . . . . . . . . . . . . 9
    Dietary Fiber . . . . . . . . . . . . . . . . . . . . . . . . . . . 15
    Vitamin A and Vitamin C . . . . . . . . . . . . . . . . 18
    Cruciferous Vegetables . . . . . . . . . . . . . . . . . . 22
    Other Dietary Factors . . . . . . . . . . . . . . . . . . . 23
    Vegetable Protein . . . . . . . . . . . . . . . . . . . . . . 23
    Vitamin D . . . . . . . . . . . . . . . . . . . . . . . . . . . . . 25
    Vitamin E . . . . . . . . . . . . . . . . . . . . . . . . . . . . . 25
    Folic Acid . . . . . . . . . . . . . . . . . . . . . . . . . . . . . 27
    Vitamin $B_6$ . . . . . . . . . . . . . . . . . . . . . . . . . . . . 28
    Iron . . . . . . . . . . . . . . . . . . . . . . . . . . . . . . . . . . 28
    Selenium . . . . . . . . . . . . . . . . . . . . . . . . . . . . . . 30
    Zinc . . . . . . . . . . . . . . . . . . . . . . . . . . . . . . . . . . 32

**Section III:**
**Alcohol, Food Additives, and**
**Natural Carcinogens** . . . . . . . . . . . . . . . . . . . . . . . 33
    Alcohol . . . . . . . . . . . . . . . . . . . . . . . . . . . . . . . 33
    Food Additives . . . . . . . . . . . . . . . . . . . . . . . . 34
    Nitrites and Nitrates . . . . . . . . . . . . . . . . . . . . 34
    Sugar . . . . . . . . . . . . . . . . . . . . . . . . . . . . . . . . 35
    Artificial Sweeteners . . . . . . . . . . . . . . . . . . . . 35
    Other Food Additives . . . . . . . . . . . . . . . . . . . 36

Natural Carcinogens............................ 36
Aflatoxin ..................................... 37
Coffee......................................... 38
Carcinogens Formed During Cooking......... 38
Summary ..................................... 40

**Section IV:**
**Dietary Guidelines for the Prevention**
**of Cancer**..................................... 41
How to Reduce the Fat and Calories
  in the Diet ................................. 42
How to Increase the Fiber in the Diet........ 49
How to Increase Foods High in Vitamin A
  and Vitamin C in the Diet ............... 51
How to Increase the Intake of Cruciferous
  Vegetables................................. 52
How to Avoid Salt-Cured and Smoked
  Foods and Foods that Might
  Cause Cancer ............................ 53
The Anti-Cancer Diet .................... 54

**References** ................................. 59
**Glossary** .................................... 67
**Index**....................................... 70

# Introduction

The news about cancer is good. At the turn of the century few people survived the disease for more than a few years. Today, three in eight persons who develop cancer will live longer than five years.[1]

These numbers are small, however, in comparison to the number of people who might never develop cancer if a few changes were made in lifestyle and dietary habits. Diet and environmental factors might be related to 80% of all cancers.[2,3] The most common fatal cancers, lung, large intestine, and breast, are directly related to either cigarette smoke or diet.[4,5] Smoking is the cause of more cancer than any other known substance. A high-fat, low-fiber diet is linked to cancer of the bowel and breast.[4,5]

The evidence supports prevention as a way to reduce cancer incidence. Prevention begins with the individual and includes healthy eating habits, moderate alcohol consumption, regular physical activity, avoidance of cigarette smoke, regular medical checkups, and minimizing exposure to pollutants in the air, water, and food. It is never too late to begin. In many cases, cancer can be avoided.

CANCER AND NUTRITION provides information on the relationships between diet and cancer prevention or cancer promotion. This book is not intended to replace the advice of a physician or an annual medical checkup. If you are concerned about your risk for cancer, discuss your diet, lifestyle, and health with a physican.

# 1
# What is Cancer?

Cancer is the uncontrolled growth and spread of abnormal cells. These cells invade and destroy surrounding tissues. By a process called metastasis, cancer cells spread through the blood and lymph systems and form new cancerous growths in other parts of the body. *(Figure 1, page 2)*

In normal circumstances, the cells of the body reproduce in an orderly manner. There is a balance between cell birth and cell death that regulates the replacement, repair, and growth of tissues. Other regulatory processes curtail excessive cell growth and control the size and shape of organs and tissues.

Normal cells can convert to abnormal cancer cells. Cancer cells reproduce more rapidly than normal cells and ignore normal regulations of when, how, and where to grow. Normal cells are more concerned with function than growth; cancer cells are more concerned with growth than function. Cancer cells exhibit no "social responsibility", they serve no useful purpose, and they cause damage by invading or pushing aside surrounding tissues.

The causes of cancer are not well-understood. It is suspected that there are two stages in the develop-

**Metastasis: The Spread of Cancer Cells**

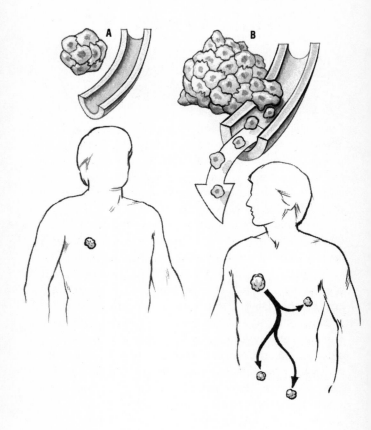

**Figure 1.** Cancer cells spread through the blood and lymph systems by a process called metastasis and form new cancerous growths in other parts of the body. Often, these secondary tumors are the cause of death.

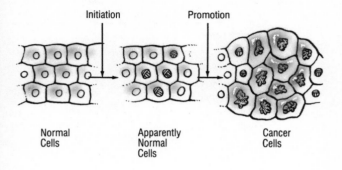

**Figure 2.** The two stages of cancer growth are initiation and promotion.

ment of cancer: an initiation phase and a promotion phase. *(Figure 2)*

In the initiation phase, the normal cell is exposed to a cancer-causing substance, called a mutagen or a carcinogen, which converts it to an abnormal cell. During the promotion phase, the abnormal cell multiplies. This latter phase can last for years and often cancer growth continues undetected for 20 to 30 years.[1]

The body must be exposed to certain conditions during both the initiation phase and the promotion phase for cancer to develop. Unless the abnormal cells formed during the initiation phase are exposed to "tumor promoters" during the promotion phase,

| Table 1 | Common Dietary Initiators and Promoters of Cancer | |
|---------|---------|---------|
| | **Initiators** | **Promoters** |
| | Nitrosamine | Saccharine |
| | Benzo(a)pyrenes in Barbecued Meats | Excess Dietary Fat |
| | | Coroton Oil |
| | Pesticides (Malathion, Parathion, Kepone, DDT) | Citrus Oil |
| | | 12-0-tetradecanoyl-phorbol-13-acetate |
| | Aflatoxin | |
| | Polychlorinated biphenyl (PCB) | High Temperatures (43-45 Degrees Centigrade) |
| | Polyvinylchloride (PVC) | Alcohol |
| | Certain Heavy Metals Such As Lead, Mercury, and Arsenic Compounds | Surface Active Agents (Sodium Lauryl Sulfate) |
| | Tannic Acid | Some Herbs, Streptomyces |

it is unlikely that cancer will develop.[1-3] In addition, the health of the immune system, the body's defense against infection and disease, might be important in protecting the body from the development and growth of abnormal cells.[6] *(Table 1)*

Many substances in food initiate and promote cancer. Nitrosamines, food additives that are found in processed meats, are initiators of cancer. Alcohol does not initiate cancer, but it does promote the growth of pre-existing cancer cells.

While the diet includes substances that encourage the growth of cancer, it also offers protection from

| Table 2 | Dietary Factors and Cancer | |
|---------|----------------------------|---|
| | **Cause Cancer** | **Prevent Cancer** |
| | High Fat Intake | High Fiber Diet |
| | Alcohol | Vegetable Intake |
| | Nitrites/Nitrates/Nitrosamines | Vitamin A/Beta Carotene |
| | Fungus Toxin (Aflatoxin) | |
| | Cooking | Vitamin C |
| | Saccharin Cyclamates | Vitamin E |
| | | Selenium |

the disease. A diet low in fat and alcohol, and high in fiber, vitamin A and vitamin C, and the trace mineral selenium inhibits the initiation and discourages the promotion of several types of cancer. *(Table 2)*

Nutritional deficiencies, as well as dietary excesses, exert an influence on cancer growth. It is estimated that diet accounts for up to 70% of all cancers and is the most influential environmental cause of cancer in addition to smoking.[7] The National Academy of Sciences states that ". . . cancer of most major sites is influenced by dietary patterns."[8] There is much a person can do to prevent the initiation and promotion of cancer.

# 2
# Nutrition and the Prevention of Cancer

There are no dietary guidelines that will guarantee protection from developing cancer. However, enough evidence exists to offer recommendations about nutrition habits that might reduce a person's risk for the disease. These recommendations are consistent with general dietary recommendations for good health. They also are similar to the dietary guidelines for the prevention and control of other degenerative diseases, such as cardiovascular disease and diabetes.[9]

A combination of the dietary recommendations for the prevention of cancer, proposed by the National Research Council and The American Cancer Society's Medical and Scientific Committee, provide guidelines for the total diet.[8,10] The risk for cancer is related to the overall quality of the diet. *(Table 3, page 8)*

## Ideal Body Weight

People who maintain an ideal body weight live longer and are less likely to develop cancer.[11,12] Low-calorie diets also might reduce the incidence of tumor formation, although this might be caused

| Table 3 | Dietary Recommendations for the Prevention of Cancer |
|---------|------------------------------------------------------|

1. Maintain Ideal Body Weight
2. Reduce Fat Intake
3. Increase High Fiber Foods
4. Frequently Include Foods Rich In Vitamin A And Vitamin C
5. Frequently Include Cruciferous Vegetables
6. Be Moderate In The Consumption Of Alcoholic Beverages
7. Be Moderate In The Consumption Of Salt-Cured, Smoked, And Nitrite-Cured Foods
8. Minimize The Consumption Of Contaminated Foods. Certain Non-Nutritive Substances In Foods, Whether Naturally Or Inadvertently Introduced During Growing, Processing, And Storage, Can Pose A Potential Risk For Cancer.
9. Minimize The Consumption Of Foods That Contain Mutagens, Such As the Methylxanthines In Tea And Coffee And The Bioamines In Cheese And Mushrooms.

more by the reduction in fat and sugar than by the reduction in total calories. People who are 20% or more above their ideal body weight are more likely to develop certain cancers, such as cancers of the uterus, gallbladder, kidney, prostate, cervix, stomach, colon, and breast.[11-13] In one study, overweight men who consumed a high-fat diet that contained milk, cheese, eggs, and meat had almost a four times greater risk for prostate cancer than men who consumed a low-fat diet and maintained a normal weight.[12]

To reduce the risk for developing cancer, a person should maintain his or her weight within the normal range by consuming a diet of nutrient-dense foods and moderate calories. Excess dieting, compulsive avoidance of food, or erratic food intake to control weight are not healthy alternatives to obesity. These eating behaviors might result in nutrient deficiencies and strain health.

## Dietary Fat and Cholesterol

Reducing the intake of dietary fat would do more for a person's health than any other dietary change. Many studies report that a diet high in fat is strongly linked to, and perhaps causes, a high incidence of cancer of the breast, ovaries, uterus, colon, and prostate.[13-19] A low-fat diet results in low incidence of cancer.

Americans consume about 42% of their calories from fat and rank high in comparison with most nations for incidence of cancer.[3] The incidence of colon cancer was low in Japan. However, as dietary habits changed to reflect western eating styles, which are high in fat and low in fiber, the incidence of colon cancer increased.[13,14] The fact that incidence of cancers of the breast, colon, and prostate are low in some countries implies that these diseases can be prevented.

No dietary component contributes more calories for its weight than fat. At nine calories per gram, a tablespoon of salad dressing supplies more calories than nine cups of tossed green salad. A serving of fried chicken contains over one-third more calories than a serving of broiled chicken. Nonfat milk contains half the calories of its fatty whole milk counter-

9

| Table 4 | The Fat Content of Chicken: Fried And Roasted | | |
| --- | --- | --- | --- |
| **Chicken Breast** | | **Fat Per Serving (4 Oz.)** | **Percent Of Calories From Fat** |
| Roasted, w/o skin | | 4 grams | 19% |
| Fried, w/o skin | | 5 | 23 |
| Roasted, w/skin | | 9 | 36 |
| Fried (flour coated), w/skin | | 10 | 36 |
| Fried (batter dipped), w/skin | | 15 | 46 |

part. *(Table 4)* These high calorie, but low nutrient contributions, might encourage the likelihood for obesity and, therefore, cancer. A reduction in dietary fat intake would help maintain ideal body weight.

The link between dietary fat intake and cancer goes beyond calories. A high-fat diet stimulates the production and excretion of cholesterol and bile into the intestine and might alter the type and amount of bacteria that are present. Bile is essential for the breakdown and digestion of fats and cholesterol. In the presence of excess dietary fat, however, the altered bacteria produce compounds from the excess bile. These compounds promote colon cancer.[8,13-17] This is supported by findings that greater amounts of intestinal bacteria that convert bile to cancer-causing compounds are found in people who consume fatty meats than in those who consume a vegetarian diet.[18,20] Colon cancer rates are lower in members of certain religious groups who consume a low-fat,

**Table 5**  A Comparison Of Fat And Fiber In Dried Beans, Beef, And Cheese

| Food | Serving | Calories | Fat (Grams) | Dietary Fiber (Grams) |
|------|---------|----------|-------------|------------------------|
| Dried Beans | 5/6 cup, cooked | 182 | 1 | 8 |
| Lentils | 5/6 cup, cooked | 177 | 0 | 6 |
| Soybeans | 5/6 cup, cooked | 195 | 8 | NA |
| Ground Beef | 4 oz., cooked | 324 | 23 | 0 |
| Cheddar Cheese | 1.5 oz. | 170 | 14 | 0 |

high-fiber vegetarian diet than in the rest of the American population.[19]

A high intake of dietary fat also is linked to breast cancer. In countries where the consumption of fat is low, the incidence of breast cancer is a fraction of that found in the United States.[19,20] People in the United States who consume a low-fat diet have less risk for developing breast cancer than people on a normal high-fat diet.[20] When the diets of women with breast cancer and and the diets of healthy women are compared, the women with cancer eat more high-fat foods, including red meat, pork, and desserts.[8] *(Table 5)*

The reason why a high-fat diet might cause breast cancer is unclear. A high-fat diet might change hormone levels, such as estrogen, and these changes are more conducive to the development of breast cancer.[8,11,21,22]

The low incidence of cancers of the ovaries and uterus in individuals who consume a diet low in fat further supports the theory that a high-fat consumption is linked to alterations in hormone activity. The risk for ovarian cancer increases two-fold to three-fold when a woman consumes a high-fat diet.[8] Women with ovarian cancer consume more fats from whole milk, butter, and other foods from animal sources and less nonfat milk, margarine, and fish than healthy women.[23,24]

The occurrence of prostate cancer is similar to the occurrence of breast cancer. Excessive fat intake is a major contributor to prostate cancer, possibly because of fat's influence on hormone metabolism.

Westernized countries have high rates of prostate cancer as compared to countries where the people consume a low-fat diet; when those people move to the United States, their risk for developing prostate cancer increases.[3]

All forms of dietary fat are linked to cancer. The saturated fats found in foods from animal sources and the unsaturated or polyunsaturated fats in foods from plant sources and vegetable oils both increase the risk of developing cancer.[25] Vegetable oils cannot replace butter in the diet, so the total fat intake should be reduced.

Saturated fats from meat and dairy foods are linked to cancer. When people consume a diet high in fatty meats and low in fruits and vegetables the risk for cancer increases eight-fold as compared to people who eat a low-fat, high-fiber diet.[26]

The polyunsaturated fats in vegetable oils are as likely to cause cancer as saturated fats. Polyunsaturated fats are thought to reduce the risk for developing cardiovascular disease, but they cannot substitute for saturated fats without increasing a person's risk for cancer.

Dietary polyunsaturated fats are incorporated into cell membranes in the body. The fats are susceptible to damage, called oxidation, by highly reactive compounds. These highly reactive compounds are called free radicals and are formed from air pollution, radiation, and the natural metabolism of proteins. Once damaged, the altered polyunsaturated fat can trigger a chain reaction that causes damage to other fats and can damage or destroy cells and tissues. This process might cause cancer.

Another type of fat that is linked to cancer is trans-fatty acids found in margarine and shortening. These fats are found sparingly in nature, but levels can be high in hydrogenated vegetable oils.[27] Trans-fatty acids are absorbed, but might not be used as readily by the cells. When they are used they act more like saturated fats than polyunsaturated fats. Trans-fatty acids might impair cell function and they could be involved in the development of cancer.[28,29]

Cholesterol is also suspected in the link between dietary fat and cancer. When people with cardiovascular disease take a medication that increases the excretion of cholesterol, the incidence of colon cancer increases. This suggests that high concentrations of cholesterol in the lower bowel might increase the risk for developing colon cancer.[30] Smokers, a group at high risk for lung cancer, might increase this risk by consuming a diet high in cholesterol.[31] *(Table 6)*

| Table 6 | Cholesterol Content Of Selected Foods | |
|---------|--------------------------------------|---|
| **Portion** | **Food** | **Average Cholesterol (mg)** |
| 1 | egg | 250 |
| 1 ounce | liver, cooked | 125 |
| 1 ounce | shrimp, cooked | 40 |
| 1 cup | milk (whole) | 30 |
| 1 ounce | beef, pork, lamb, crab, lobster, cooked | 25 |
| 1 ounce | poultry, cooked | 25 |
| 1 ounce | fish, clams, oysters, cooked | 20 |
| 1 teaspoon | butter | 10 |
| 1 teaspoon | mayonnaise | 5 |
| 1 teaspoon | margarine, vegetable oil | 0 |
| 1 cup | legumes, cooked | 0 |
| 1 cup | rice, oats, pasta, cooked; fruit; vegetable | 0 |

Compounds that act as tumor promoters might be produced when dietary fats turn rancid. The consumption of vegetable oils and other dietary fats that contain some rancid fats can expose the intestine to cancer-causing substances.[32]

A reduction in dietary cholesterol and all fats would decrease the risk for developing several types of cancer.

## Dietary Fiber

The combination of a high-fat diet with a low intake of fiber is linked to cancer of the colon.[33] In countries where the consumption of fiber foods is low, people have as much as eight times the incidence of colon cancer as people in countries where fiber intake is high.[34,35] When people who consume ample amounts of dietary fiber move to the United States and consume a low-fiber, high-fat diet, their rate of colon cancer increases.[13,36-38] People with colon cancer consume less fiber than people who are cancer-free.[8]

Fiber also might affect the incidence of breast cancer. Women who are vegetarians and consume a fiber-rich diet, 28 grams each day, excrete more estrogen than women who consume the typical American diet containing 12 grams of fiber daily. The increased removal of estrogen suggests that less estrogen is reabsorbed.[39] Vegetarian women also have lower blood levels of other hormones.[22] These changes in estrogen and other hormones are associated with a reduced risk of breast cancer.

The effects of fiber on estrogen levels complement the effects of a low-fat diet, which protects an individual from breast cancer. Vegetarian women consume a diet containing 30% fat and have a low incidence of breast cancer, compared to women who eat meat and consume over 40% of their calories as fat. As with colon cancer, the combined effects of a low-

15

fat, high-fiber diet are a key element in breast cancer prevention.

There are many types of fiber and different fibers are found in different foods. Not all types of fiber help prevent cancer. Cellulose is the type of fiber found in wheat bran. Hemicellulose, another form of fiber, is found in whole grain cereals, and lignin is found in whole grains, fruits, and vegetables. Pectin is found in apples and other fruits. Gums, such as guar gum, are found in beans, oats, fruits, and vegetables. *(Table 7)*

The insoluble fibers, such as cellulose or wheat bran, appear to be the best protectors against cancer. The insoluble fibers bind to water, increase the bulk in the intestine, and leave less room for harmful cancer-causing substances to act. In addition, these fibers dilute the contents of the intestine and reduce the strength of any cancer-causing substances that might be present. Fiber also speeds the movement of undigested foods, bacteria, and other wastes through the intestines and reduces the time cancerous substances are in contact with the intestinal wall. Cellulose and other insoluble fibers might alter the type and activity of bacteria in the intestine and reduce their ability to produce cancer-causing compounds. Finally, some cancer-causing compounds are formed from bile. Fiber binds to bile and discourages its conversion to harmful substances.[40]

Other types of cancer prevention have been attributed to fiber. Pectin decreases the production of certain fatty acids that are known to accelerate the growth of cancer cells in the bowel.[41] Lignin, a fiber in some vegetables, has antioxidant properties. Lignin

16

| Table 7 | Classification of Dietary Fiber | |
|---|---|---|
| | **Type of Fiber** | **Function** |
| | Gums (guar gum, locust bean gum) | Slow emptying of stomach<br>Bind bile acids |
| | Mucilages (plant seeds) | Slow emptying of stomach<br>Bind bile acids |
| | Algae and seaweeds | Slow emptying of stomach<br>Bind bile acids |
| | Pectin | Slow emptying of stomach<br>Bind bile acids |
| | Hemicellulose (grains, vegetables) | Hold water and increase bulk of stool<br>Might bind bile acids |
| | Cellulose (grains, vegetables) | Hold water<br>Might bind trace minerals and reduce their absorption |
| | Lignin (woody portion of plants) | Antioxidant<br>Might bind trace minerals |

might protect a cell from damage by free radicals and might protect against some forms of cancer.[3,13] Another benefit of fiber in the prevention of cancer is that it contains no calories, but it does contribute bulk to the diet. A person can eat more food and consume less calories when the foods are high in fiber. This helps maintain weight and eliminate hunger.

The fiber issue is not clear cut. A low-fiber diet is often a high-fat diet. Since dietary fat is strongly linked to cancer and obesity it is hard to separate the effects of these two dietary components.[11] This close association between fat and fiber emphasizes the importance of the entire diet, not just one nutrient or component, in the prevention of cancer.

## Vitamin A and Vitamin C

**Vitamin A:** A diet that contains ample amounts of vitamin A, and its form found in plant sources, beta carotene, is associated with a reduced risk for developing some cancers including cancer of the mouth, larynx, esophagus (throat), breast, cervix, bladder, and lungs.[42-44] Diets that are low in vitamin A or beta carotene increase a person's risk for cancer.[44]

Vitamin A comes in two dietary forms. Retinol, the vitamin A found in foods from animal sources such as liver, milk, and eggs, is the preformed, active form of the vitamin. The carotenoids are the provitamin form of vitamin A found in plants. Of the over 400 carotenoids identified, 50 can be converted to retinol in the body. Beta carotene is the most common and most active carotenoid. *(Table 8)*

The two-step process in the development of cancer includes an initiation and a promotion phase. (See page 3) Vitamin A and beta carotene play an inhibitory role in both of these phases.

Although how vitamin A works is not well understood, several theories have been proposed.

| Table 8 | Beta Carotene Content of Selected Foods | |
| --- | --- | --- |
| **Vegetable** | **Serving Size** | **Beta Carotene (micrograms)** |
| Collard greens | 1 cup cooked | 8,892 |
| Spinach | 1 cup raw | 2,676 |
| Squashes: | | |
| butternut | 1 cup | 7,872 |
| acorn | 1 cup | 1,722 |
| yellow | 1 cup | 636 |
| zucchini | 1 cup | 432 |
| Cataloupe | 1/2 | 5,544 |
| Carrots | 1 raw | 4,758 |
| Beet greens | 1 cup cooked | 4,440 |
| Broccoli | 1 cup cooked | 2,320 |
| Apricots | 1 | 1,734 |
| Prunes | 1 cup | 1,302 |
| Peaches | 1 large | 1,218 |
| Watermelon | 1 cup | 564 |

Vitamin A or beta carotene might

- inhibit the growth of abnormal cells so that cancer tissue is unable to form;
- alter immune function and improve the body's defense against abnormal cell growth;
- strengthen cell membranes and make them less vulnerable to attack or damage;
- or alter cell production so that abnormal cells are less likely to form.[44]

Vitamin A is necessary for the normal growth and development of epithelial tissues. These tissues line all surfaces of the body, inside and outside. Examples of epithelial tissue include the outer surface of the eye; the skin; the lining of the lungs, colon, stomach, prostate, cervix, and uterus; and the mucous-lining of the throat and mouth. An inadequate intake of vitamin A might affect the health, growth, or maintenance of these tissues and increase the likelihood of cancer.[45,46] Epithelial cancers account for over one-half of all cancers in men and women.[47]

People who consume diets that contain several servings of foods rich in vitamin A or beta carotene each day are less likely to develop cancer of the lungs, colon, stomach, prostate, and cervix.[13] Numerous studies have confirmed the anticancer effects of vitamin A and show that when vitamin A or beta carotene intake is high, risk for cancers of the lung, bladder, mouth, larynx, breast, cervix, and throat are low.[48] In addition, cancer rates are highest in people with low amounts of vitamin A in their blood.[11]

Beta carotene might reduce the risk for developing lung cancer. Lung cancer rates are lower in smokers who consume a diet high in fruits and vegetables than in smokers who avoid fruit and vegetables. When the intake of beta carotene is low, the incidence of lung cancer in smokers increases.[49]

The recommended dietary allowance (RDA) for vitamin A might not be adequate to reduce a person's risk for cancer.[48] The adult RDA of 4,000 IU to 5,000 IU is designed to protect against the development of night blindness, which is the classic vitamin A deficiency disease. Larger doses for this fat-soluble vitamin, between 10,000 IU and 25,000 IU, have been suggested to decrease the risk of cancer.[48] Because vitamin A can be toxic, large doses on a routine basis are discouraged. Beta carotene is not toxic. Long-term large doses can be taken with no apparent harmful effects other than a temporary yellowing of the skin that subsides when the dose is reduced.

The link between foods rich in vitamin A/beta carotene and the inhibition of cancer is strong. Other anticancer substances in these foods, such as fiber, however, might contribute to their effectiveness.

Foods high in vitamin A/beta carotene include dark green and orange vegetables such as carrots, broccoli, winter squash, sweet potatoes, pumpkin, and spinach; apricots, cantaloupe, peaches, and watermelon; liver; and some dairy products such as cheese & fortified nonfat milk.

**Vitamin C:** People who consume several servings each day of vitamin C-rich fruits and vegetables are less likely to develop cancer of the stomach and throat. Low vitamin C consumption is linked with an increased risk for these cancers.[50-53]

Nitrosamines are cancer-causing substances found in a variety of foods and in cigarette smoke.[54] They are also formed in the stomach from nitrites, which are additives in processed meats. Although vitamin C cannot halt the cancer-causing effects of nitrosamines in foods, it can inhibit the conversion of nitrites to nitrosamines in the stomach and reduce the risk of developing stomach cancer.[44] In areas where the intake of vitamin C foods is low, the risk for cancer of the stomach is high.[50,51,55]

Vitamin C might reduce the risk for developing bladder cancer. In recurrent bladder infections compounds related to nitrosamines are converted to cancer-causing substances. Vitamin C blocks the formation of these substances and might protect against bladder cancer.[56]

A low intake of vitamin C might increase a person's risk for developing colon cancer. Vitamin C might reduce the formation of cancer-causing substances in the intestine that could lead to cancer.[57]

There are several ways vitamin C might prevent cancer. The vitamin might improve the cell's resistance to damage, enhance the immune system and strengthen the body's defense against disease, or protect cells from damage by oxidation. The latter effect of vitamin C is a result of the vitamin's antioxidant role in the deactivation of free radicals.[11]

Vitamin C is found in vegetables and fruits. Good dietary sources include citrus fruits, strawberries, broccoli, cantaloupe, potatoes, and asparagus. Meats, eggs, dairy foods, and grains are poor sources of vitamin C. *(Table 9, page 23)*

## Cruciferous Vegetables

Vegetables that belong to the cruciferous family include cabbage, Brussels sprouts, kohlrabi, cauliflower, and broccoli. Frequent consumption of these vegetables might reduce the risk of some types of cancer, especially stomach, colon, and respiratory tract cancer. The protective effect is associated with non-nutritive substances in these vegetables called

| Table 9 | Vitamin C Content of Selected Fruits and Vegetables | | |
|---------|--------------------|--------------|----------------|
| | Food | Serving Size[b] | Vitamin C (mg) |
| | Brussels Sprouts | 1/2 cup | 68 |
| | Strawberries | 3/4 cup | 66 |
| | Orange Juice | 1/2 cup | 60 |
| | Broccoli | 1/2 cup | 52 |
| | Cantaloupe | 1/4 | 32 |
| | Asparagus | 1/2 cup | 19 |
| | Potato (Baked) | 1 Small | 15 |
| | Bananas | 1/2 Medium | 6 |
| | Corn | 1/3 Cup | 4 |
| | Yogurt | 1 Cup | 2 |

indoles.[8,10,21] The added benefit of cruciferous vegetables is they also contain vitamin A and vitamin C.


## Other Dietary Factors

Other substances in foods inhibit the development of cancer in addition to low fat, fiber, vitamin A and vitamin C, and the indoles in cruciferous vegetables. These include vegetable protein, vitamin D, vitamin E, folic acid, vitamin $B_6$, iron, selenium, and zinc. Frequent inclusion in the daily diet of foods that contain these vitamins, minerals, and other compounds will help reduce a person's risk for cancer.

**Vegetable protein:** Protein from vegetable sources might reduce the risk for cancer. Vegetarians have a lower incidence of cancer than people who consume a diet of animal protein. Although the preventive effects on cancer are poorly understood, a diet that derives most of its protein from vegetable sources might contain compounds that inhibit the growth of cancer.

Protease inhibitors are compounds found in vegetable sources of protein, such as soybeans corn, beans, and rice. These compounds might block the formation of some types of cancer, including liver, breast, and colon cancer.[61] Evidence shows that if one-third to one-half of the day's allotment of protein comes from dried beans and peas the risk for developing cancer might be reduced.[61] These foods are high in fiber, which is another dietary aid in the prevention of cancer.

In contrast, evidence suggests that a diet that provides most of its protein from animal sources, especially red meats, increases a person's risk for developing cancer. People who consume a large amount of animal protein from milk, cheese, eggs, and meat might have four times the risk for prostate cancer as people who consume most of their protein from vegetable sources.[12]

A diet high in animal fat and protein is linked to an increased risk for pancreatic cancer. Animal protein and fat might act as co-carcinogens to increase the rate of growth and spread of cancer.[58]

Illness and death from lymphoma, which is cancer of the lymph system, is linked to the consumption of animal protein, especially beef protein.[59] These cancers are lower in people who consume mostly vegetable protein. In countries where the consumption of protein is changing from mostly vegetable protein to mostly animal protein, the death rate from colon cancer also is increasing.[60]

It is difficult to separate the affects of animal protein from animal fat. Some of the evidence linking meat protein with cancer might be a result of the high-fat, low-fiber aspects of these foods. Vegetable protein foods are also high fiber foods and fiber protects against some types of cancer. Protein might have an independent affect on cancer, however, since a high animal protein diet might affect the initiation phase of cancer formation and stimulate cancer growth. A diet that contains vegetable protein might be a prudent step in the prevention of cancer.[8]

**Vitamin D:** Vitamin D might be linked to the prevention of cancer of the breast and colon and the vitamin might slow the growth of some types of cancer.[62,63] Rates of colon cancer increase in areas where people have limited exposure to the sun. Since vitamin D can be produced by skin cells in the presence of sunlight, this association between colon cancer and sun exposure suggests that inadequate synthesis of vitamin D is involved in the progression of colon cancer. This association is further supported by evidence that the risk for developing colon cancer increases as the dietary intake of vitamin D decreases.[63]

**Vitamin E:** Vitamin E's function as an antioxidant is its primary link in the prevention of cancer. Vitamin E prevents the formation of free radicals, highly reactive compounds that damage cells and tissues, and other compounds suspected to be carcinogens (cancer-causing substances).

Free radicals attack fats in cell membranes and alter the membrane's structure or function. This damage sets up a chain reaction that destroys surrounding fats. The cell membrane is damaged and the cell might die. Vitamin E protects fats in the body from free radical damage and might discourage the formation of abnormal cells.

Preliminary evidence shows vitamin E might inhibit the growth of cancer.[64] This fat-soluble vitamin reduces the formation of nitrosamines from dietary nitrites and might reduces the risk for development of stomach cancer.[60] Vitamin E also might assist selenium, a mineral that inhibits the development of cancer, when it is present in the diet.[65]

The daily requirement for vitamin E is in proportion to the amount of polyunsaturated fats in the diet: the greater the intake of vegetable oils, nuts, and other fats, the more vitamin E is needed to protect these fats from damage.

Vitamin E is found in foods of both plant and animal sources. Vegetable oils and seed oils are the best sources. Vitamin E is actually a family of compounds called the tocopherols. Alpha tocopherol is the most active in body processes. The alpha tocopherol content varies between vegetable oils, but safflower oil contains the highest amount of this form of vitamin E. Whole grains are good sources of vitamin E, but the vitamin is lost in the milling and bleaching of refined grains. The vitamin E content of vegetable oils also declines when they are refined and bleached. The byproducts of this process contain so much vitamin E that they are used in making vitamin E supplements.[66] *(Table 10)*

| Table 10 | Vitamin E Content of Selected Foods | | |
|----------|------|---------------|------------------------|
| | Food | Serving Size | Vitamin E mg/serving |
| | Wheat germ oil | 1 tbsp | 39.0 |
| | Corn oil, hydrogenated | 1 tbsp | 15.8 |
| | Soybean oil, unhydrogenated | 1 tbsp | 15.2 |
| | Corn oil | 1 tbsp | 15.0 |
| | Safflower oil | 1 tbsp | 8.8 |
| | Wheat germ | 1 oz | 3.8 |
| | Oatmeal, uncooked | 1/4 c | 1.9 |
| | Salmon, broiled | 3 oz | 1.5 |
| | Navy beans, dry | 1/2 c | 1.5 |
| | Peas, fresh | 1/2 c | 1.5 |
| | Apple | 1 medium | 0.7 |
| | Bread, whole wheat | 1 slice | 0.6 |
| | Banana | 1 medium | 0.5 |

**Folic acid:** Folic acid is a member of the B vitamin family. The primary function of folic acid is to maintain the genetic code of cells and regulate normal cell division and growth. A folic acid deficiency causes damage to cells that resembles the initial stage of cancer.[67]

Preliminary evidence shows that folic acid might prevent the conversion of abnormal cells to cancer cells and might convert damaged cells back to normal ones.[68]

Surveys show that the folic acid content of the American diet is approximately half of the recommended daily intake.[69] The best dietary sources of folic acid are dark green leafy vegetables such as spinach, chard, romaine lettuce, and broccoli. Unfortunately, these are not foods commonly chosen in the daily diet. In addition, the vitamin is easily destroyed by heat and processing. If food is improperly stored, overcooked, or reheated, or if the cooking water is discarded, little or no folic acid will be present by the time the food is eaten. *(Table 11, page 29)*

**Vitamin B$_6$:** Vitamin B$_6$ helps strengthen the immune system. The body might have more resistance to cancer when vitamin B$_6$ is present in ample amounts.[70] Vitamin B$_6$ also might protect against the initiation of cancer.[71]

The daily need for vitamin B$_6$ is proportionate to the amount of protein in the diet. As the consumption of meats, chicken, and other protein-rich foods increases so does the need for vitamin B$_6$. Good dietary sources of this B vitamin include lean meat, chicken, fish, soybeans and dried beans, peanuts, walnuts, bananas, cabbage, cauliflower, potatoes, and whole grain breads and cereals.

Vitamin B$_6$ is lost during the cooking, freezing, and canning of foods and in the processing of refined grains. A diet that contains convenience foods, refined white breads and rice, sugary foods, and fats might not supply adequate amounts of vitamin B$_6$.[72] National surveys show that American diets are low in this vitamin.[73,74]

**Iron:** An iron deficiency might increase a person's risk for cancer.[60] Adequate iron intake is necessary

| Table 11 | Folic Acid Content of Selected Foods | |
|---|---|---|
| **Food** | | **Amount** |
| **Excellent Sources (>100 mg)** | | |
| Chickpeas, canned | | 1 cup |
| Spinach, cooked | | 1 cup |
| Orange juice | | 1 cup |
| Beets, cooked | | 1 cup |
| Wheat germ, toasted | | 1/4 c |
| Parsley, raw | | 1 Tbsp |
| Pinto beans, cooked | | 1 cup |
| Spinach, raw, packed | | 1 cup |
| Broccoli, cooked | | 1 spear |
| **Good Sources (>75 mg)** | | |
| Romaine lettuce, 1 cup | | 1 cup |
| Parsnips, raw | | 1 cup |
| Asparagus, raw | | 1 cup |
| Lima beans, cooked | | 1 cup |
| Peas, frozen | | 1 cup |
| **Fair Sources (>25 mg)** | | |
| Kale, raw | | 1 cup |
| Orange | | 1 medium |
| Brussels Sprouts, cooked | | 1 cup |
| Collards, raw | | 1 cup |
| Tomatoes, raw | | 1 medium |
| Grapefruit juice | | 1 cup |
| Turnip greens, raw | | 1 cup |
| Avocado | | 1/2 medium |
| Rutabagas, cooked & mashed | | 1 cup |
| Green beans, cooked | | 1 cup |
| Cauliflower, cooked | | 1 cup |
| Cantaloupe | | 1/4 medium |
| Banana | | 1 |

for the proper function of the immune system, which might explain the link between this mineral and cancer. Iron deficiency also might increase the risk for stomach cancer.[60]

Iron deficiency is common in women, children, infants, the elderly, minorities, and adolescents.[75] Because the diet supplies about 6 mg of iron for each 1,000 calories, a woman should consume 3,000 calories to meet her RDA of 18mg. The average calorie intake for a woman is between 1,600 and 2,000 calories. The Food and Nutrition Board states that it is unlikely that a woman can obtain the recommended iron intake from normal food consumption.[76] Supplements might be necessary.

**Selenium:** Selenium is a trace mineral that might be important in the prevention of cancer. Increased intake of selenium reduces the risk for cancer in animals and it is suspected to do the same in people. For example, when animals are fed selenium-fortified water, the incidence of cancer growth declines from 82% to 10%.[77]

People who live in areas where the selenium content of the soil is poor have higher rates for cancer of the digestive tract, lungs, breast, and lymph system than people who live in areas where the soil is selenium-rich.[78] When the selenium intake of people is studied in different countries, those people who consume a high-selenium diet are less likely to develop cancer than people in countries where the selenium content of the diet is poor.[79]

Blood levels of selenium are low in people with cancer and people with very low selenium levels have twice the risk for cancer as those with high selenium levels.[80-82] Low selenium levels are found in people with Hodgkin's disease, leukemia, and cancer of the breast, lymph system, stomach and intestine, colon, bladder and genital tract, and skin.[80-82]

Selenium might protect against cancer in several ways. Selenium is an antioxidant nutrient and apparently prevents cancer by protecting cell membranes from damage by free radicals[82,83] In addition to its effectiveness as an antioxidant, selenium also might stimulate the immune system and strengthen the body's defense against disease.[84] This mineral also protects against the toxic effects of some metals. Selenium detoxifies cadmium and mercury, two minerals known to cause cancer.[8]

The selenium content of foods depends on the selenium content of the soil in which they are grown. Plants do not need selenium and can thrive in selenium-depleted soil. Animals and people who consume these plants do require selenium and are at increased risk for a deficiency when the diet consists mostly of selenium-low plant foods.

In the United States, wheat used for breads and pasta is often grown in regions where the soil is rich in selenium. Vegetables can vary in their selenium content. Lean meats and seafood are good sources of this mineral.

Selenium is available in supplements as the organic forms, such as selenomethionine or selenocysteine and the inorganic form, which is sodium selenite. These two forms are used differently by the body and might have different effects on the development or inhibition of cancer. The organic forms are most important for health. The inorganic form of selenium might be toxic and might promote cancer when taken in large doses.[85,86]

**Zinc:** Zinc is required for the normal formation and regulation of the genetic code within each cell, the maintenance of a healthy immune system, and for healing of tissues.[87]

Zinc also might reduce a person's risk for developing cancer. People with lung cancer have low amounts of zinc in their blood and cancer might progress more rapidly in zinc-deficient cancer patients. This observation has been linked to zinc's role in the maintenance of the immune system.[88] People with a reduced resistance to infection, which is a symptom of a poorly functioning immune system, often have low levels of zinc in their blood. When zinc-rich foods are added to the diet resistance to disease improves.[89] Low levels of zinc also are found in people with prostate cancer.[90]

Whereas adequate intake of zinc might be important in the prevention of cancer, large doses of zinc might inhibit the immune system and increase the risk for infection and disease.[91]

The best dietary sources of zinc include lean meat, oysters, whole grain breads and cereals, and low-fat milk.

# 3
# Alcohol, Food Additives, and Natural Carcinogens

## Alcohol

Alcohol has been associated with cancers of the mouth, esophagus, colon, pharynx, and larynx.[92,94] The combined effects of tobacco and alcohol are strongly linked to cancer development. A recent study found an association between alcohol and breast cancer. Women who consumed alcoholic beverages had more than twice the risk of breast cancer when compared to women who abstained.[95]

How alcohol contributes to cancer risk is not well-understood, but several possible roles have been identified. Alcohol might be a carcinogen or it might enhance the cancer-causing effects of another carcinogen. As a solvent, it might facilitate the transport of carcinogens into susceptible tissues. Alcohol also might produce compounds in the body that activate carcinogens.[8]

One substance known to convert substances in the body to carcinogens is cytochrome P-450, found in the liver. Alcohol increases the level of cytochrome P-450 and is believed to be linked to the risk of certain cancers in alcoholics.[96]

Many alcoholic beverages contain other substances that might be carcinogenic. Beer consumption, but not alcohol consumption, is directly correlated with colon cancer: the greater the intake of beer, the greater the likelihood of colon cancer.[8,21]

Alcohol abuse is also associated with a suppression of the immune system, a factor that might make a person more susceptible to cancer.[8,60] Alcoholics are known for their poor food intake and poor nutritional status. Alcohol interferes with the absorption of some nutrients and raises requirements for other nutrients. Alcoholics often have low levels of vitamin A and vitamin C, folic acid, many B vitamins, zinc, and selenium.[97] Deficiencies of these vitamins and minerals are associated with an increased risk for cancer. (See pages 18, 27, 28, 30, 32)

## Food Additives

**Nitrites and Nitrates:** The dietary recommendations established by the American Cancer Society suggest that salt-cured, salt-pickled, and smoked foods be reduced or eliminated from the diet. The harmful effects of these foods are attributed to the nitrites used in processing.[10]

Nitrites and nitrates are food additives used to preserve and color processed meats such as bacon, luncheon meats, and cured meats. These compounds also occur in nature, especially in beets, celery, lettuce, spinach, radishes, and rhubarb. Nitrates can be converted to nitrites by bacteria found in saliva. Nitrites then combine with other substances found in the stomach and form cancer-causing substances called nitrosamines. In areas of the world where exposure to these substances is great, there is an increased incidence of cancers of the stomach and esophagus.[8,98]

Cigarettes are high in nitrosamines and the use of nitrogen fertilizers has increased the amount of nitrosamines in the water supply. A diet high in vitamin C and vitamin E can reduce the formation in the stomach of nitrosamines from nitrites.[60]

**Sugar:** A diet high in sugar is linked to increased risk for developing cancer of the breast and bowel.[99,100] Although these diets also are associated with reduced fiber intake, increased fat consumption, and excess calorie intake, the sugar might exert an independent effect on the incidence of cancer. A high-fat, high-sugar diet, which is characteristic of the average American diet, might have a combined effect on increasing the risk for cancer.[99,100]

**Artificial Sweeteners:** Many people turn to artificial sweeteners to satisfy their sweet tooth while reducing their calories. However, the safety of these non-nutritive sweeteners has been questioned. Cyclamates were banned in 1970 after studies showed an increase in bladder tumors.[8]

A similar story is true for saccharin. Experimental studies on animals show that saccharin, given at high doses, produces urinary tract tumors.[60] This sweetener promotes the action of other carcinogens in the bladder. Saccharin use has increased since cyclamates were banned. Saccharin might increase a person's risk for bladder cancer and as saccahrin use increases so does the risk for cancer.[8,60]

The concern over the safety of saccharin has led to an increase in the use of aspartame. This nonnutritive sweetener has only been used in Europe since 1981, and more recently in the United States. It does not appear to have negative effects on human health.[8,60]

**Other food additives:** More than 3,000 chemicals are intentionally added to foods during processing. These chemicals are added to improve color, taste, texture, and consistency and to retard spoilage.

Another 12,000 additives are added unintentionally to foods. These additives, such as vinyl chloride, migrate into foods during the growing, harvesting, packaging, or storage of the food.

Butylated hydroxytoluene (BHT) and butylated hydroxyanisole (BHA) are preservatives used to prolong the shelf-life of foods. BHT might promote the formation of tumors.[60] No cancer-promoting action has been found for BHA.

The Food and Drug Administration regulates the presence of carcinogens in foods and lists those additives that are safe on the Generally Regarded As Safe (GRAS) list. If a substance is found to cause cancer in laboratory animals it is removed from the list and banned from use. However, only a portion of the substances added to foods have been adequately tested for carcinogenicity, which is their ability to cause cancer. A diet of wholesome, fresh foods such as whole grain breads and cereals, dried beans and peas, low-fat milk, fresh fruits and vegetables, and fish, contains minor amounts of food additives, while supplying ample amounts of fiber and other dietary factors that reduce the risk for cancer.

## Natural Carcinogens

Many substances thought to cause cancer are man-made chemicals, such as pesticides, polyvinyl-chloride, and polychlorinated biphenyls (PCBs).

Many compounds that damage cells and cause cancer are natural components of foods. Many plants produce their own toxic chemicals in an effort to defend themselves against bacterial, fungal, insect, and animal predators.

One of the most well-known natural carcinogens is safrole, the primary flavor component of the bark of the sassafras tree. It was used in the production of sarsaparilla until 1960, when it was banned as a potent carcinogen.[101] Black pepper contains small amounts of safrole in addition to a large amount of a related substance, piperine; however, harmful effects are only seen when large amounts of pepper are consumed.[32,102] Other plant substances are linked to cancer. These include compounds in celery, parsnips, figs, potatoes, parsley, and other vegetables.[103,104]

There is no evidence that a moderate intake of these compounds is harmful. Vegetables that contain possible carcinogens are also high in nutritional value. Many of them also contain anticarcinogens, substances that reduce or block cancer-promoting activity. Cancer risk depends not only on exposure to carcinogenic substances but to the strength of the defense system.

A diet that contains a variety of foods safeguards against overconsumption of harmful food compounds from any one dietary source and helps guarantee adequate nutrient intake to strengthen body defenses against infection and disease.

**Aflatoxin:** A naturally-occurring carcinogen is aflatoxin. Aflatoxin is a mold that forms on corn, cottonseed, peanuts, and peanut butter when these foods are not well-preserved.[32]

Aflatoxins, the most potent liver carcinogens known, are classified as unavoidable contaminants. In the United States, a maximum allowable aflatoxin level in consumer products has been specified by the Food and Drug Administration. In regions of Africa and Asia where there is a high ingestion of aflatoxin, the incidence of liver cancer is also high.

**Coffee:** The statement that coffee or its caffeine content are linked to cancer has not been supported by research. Excess coffee consumption might be linked to a slight increase in bladder cancer incidence, but these results are not consistent between men and women and have not been substantiated by studies.[60] The link between coffee consumption and pancreatic cancer also is weak and inconclusive.[105,107] Although more research is necessary, coffee and caffeine have not been linked to an increase in cancer of any type.[107] *(Table 11a, page 39)*

## Carcinogens Formed During Cooking

While a food might not be carcinogenic, the method used to prepare it might cause changes in the food that might make it carcinogenic. Frying, barbecuing, or broiling meats and fish at high temperatures can produce cancer-promoting substances from the fats and proteins in these foods.

When meat is barbecued, the high heat in cooking and the protein and fatty portions of the meat combine to form a cancer-causing substance called benzo [a] pyrene. Exactly how much benzo [a] pyrene collects on the surface of the meat depends on the amount of fat and protein in the meat, the tempera-

| Table 11a | The Caffeine Content of Coffee | |
|---|---|---|
| Coffee (5 oz. cup) | Milligrams Caffeine Average |
| Brewed, drip method | 115 |
| Brewed, percolator | 80 |
| Instant | 65 |
| Decaffeinated, brewed | 3 |
| Decaffeinated, instant | 2 |

**Source:** FDA, Food Additive Chemistry Evaluation Branch, based on evaluations of existing literature on caffeine levels.

ture of the cooking, and the length of time the meat is exposed to the flame.

Smoked foods, such as ham, sausage, fish, or oysters, absorb the tars that are produced from the incomplete combustion of fuel. These tars contain several cancer-causing substances that are similar to the carcinogenic tars in tobacco smoke. The liquid smoke sold commercially is less hazardous.

Cancer-causing substances also have been found in other foods that are browned, such as toast and fried potatoes. Dark roasted coffee contains some potential carcinogens.[8]

## Summary

Although some dietary factors have been linked to an increased risk for cancer, that does not prove that those factors *cause* cancer. It is more likely that nutritional imbalances are coupled with other environmental hazards that might weaken the immune system and other natural body defenses. A healthy diet plays a major role in the prevention of cancer.

# 4
# Dietary Guidelines for the Prevention of Cancer

The good news about cancer is there is something each person can do to prevent it. The most important step to take in the prevention of cancer is **don't smoke,** if you smoke — **quit,** and avoid other people's cigarette smoke.

Dietary patterns that reduce a person's risk for developing cancer include:

- maintaining ideal body weight;
- reducing dietary fat;
- increasing dietary fiber;
- increasing intake of foods high in vitamin A and vitamin C;
- increasing intake of cruciferous vegetables;
- limiting intake of salt-cured, smoked, and nitrite-cured foods;
- avoiding contaminated foods;
- avoiding foods that might contain carcinogens and mutagens; and
- drinking alcohol in moderation.

These dietary recommendations can be individualized to meet the specific needs of each person. A person does not need to abandon certain dietary habits and patterns, but can adapt and adjust the

41

diet to reflect the anti-cancer recommendations while still including personal favorite foods.

It is never to late to make dietary adjustments that could save your life. Even diet changes made late in life can help prevent some forms of cancer. In addition, it is never too early to begin healthy eating habits. Except for children under one year of age, a low-fat, low-sugar diet is recommended for all age groups. The establishment of healthy eating patterns early in life is often easier than trying to change long-held habits. The consumption of a low-fat, high-fiber diet throughout life might aid in the prevention of cancer, cardiovascular disease, diabetes, hypertension, and obesity.[4,8-10]

## How To Reduce The Fat And Calories In The Diet

Reducing the consumption of fat is the most important dietary change a person can make to prevent cancer, other degenerative diseases, and obesity.[8] The current consumption of fat is approximately 42% of total calories. Fat consumption should total no more than 30% of total calories if the risk for developing cancer and other diseases is to be reduced.[8,9] *(Table 12)*

Reducing the fat in the diet does not mean reducing the flavor. A diet that contains 30% of its calories as fat can taste good, look good, and be good.

There are four guidelines to remember when reducing the fat in the diet.

1. Most of the food in the diet (two-thirds to three-quarters) should come from foods from plant sources such as fresh fruits and vegetables, whole

| Table 12 | What Is Your Daily Fat Allowance? |
| --- | --- |
| **1.** | What is your average daily calorie intake? _____ |
| **2a.** | To calculate a 30% fat allowance, multiply your average daily calorie intake by 0.3 = _____ (this provides the total number of calories that can come from fat). |
| **b.** | To calculate a 20% fat allowance, multiply your average daily calorie intake by 0.2 = _____ |
| **3.** | Divide the total number of calories that can come from fat (question 2) by 9 (there are 9 calories in each gram of fat) = _____ |
| | This is your fat allowance — in grams. |

grain breads and cereals, and dried beans and peas. These foods are high in fiber and low in fat and sugar. The fruits and vegetables are good dietary sources of vitamin A and vitamin C. A rule of thumb is three out of every four foods or three-quarters of the food on a plate should be foods from plant sources. For example, a typical breakfast might be:

Oatmeal (1 cup)
Low-fat milk (1/2 cup)
Whole wheat toast (2 slices)
Margarine (1 tsp)
Orange juice (6 ounces)

Lunch and dinner might include salads, vegetable-bean soup, spaghetti with marinara sauce, fresh fruit plate, baked potato with chives, steamed vegetables, or rolls. The selections are endless.

The only exceptions in the fruit and vegetable category are olives, avocados, and coconut. These foods are high in fat. They do not need to be eliminated from the diet, just used in moderation.

Starches are a misunderstood carbohydrate. They are not fattening and should be increased in the diet, not reduced. Most foods high in starch are also high in vitamins and minerals. If these foods are obtained from the whole grain varieties they are also high in fiber. Unless fat is added in processing, starchy foods are low in fat. Examples of starches that contain added fat include granolas, croissants, crescent rolls, flaky biscuits, and some muffins.

Desserts, doughnuts, cakes, and breakfast rolls contain some refined starch, but are high in sugar and fat. Low-fat desserts include angel food cake, gingersnaps, and some gingerbread recipes. The fat content of most recipes can be reduced by one-third to one-half with no change in taste or texture.

2. Low-fat and nonfat dairy foods should be emphasized rather than fatty dairy foods. Whole and fatty dairy foods are high in saturated fats and cholesterol and inclusion of these foods in the diet might increase a person's risk for cancer. The change from whole milk dairy foods to low-fat or nonfat should be gradual. Choose low-fat or nonfat milk, cottage cheese, cheese (partially skimmed mozzarella, swiss, or jarlsberg) or yogurt. An

ounce of cheddar cheese supplies over 70% of its calories as fat. Use low-fat dairy foods in cooking and at the table. Nonfat milk with added nonfat dry milk powder can be used to thicken soups, sauces, and gravies. Evaporated nonfat milk also can be used in recipes to replace cream and whole milk. Use nonfat yogurt instead of sour cream or mix the two to produce a dip that is lower in fat than plain sour cream. (Table 13, page 46)

3. Lean meat, poultry without the skin, and fish should be used, but no more than 6 ounces a day. Beef, pork, and other red meats, as well as whole eggs, are major sources of saturated fats and cholesterol. Choose meats that are less than 15% fat by weight, trim all visible fat from red meats, and replace red meats with poultry and fish whenever possible. Lean cuts of beef include rump and round roasts, round steaks, flank steaks, and sirloin steaks. The leanest cut of pork is ham; however, cured ham is high in salt and sodium nitrite. The Committee on Diet, Nutrition, and Cancer recommends that cured foods be avoided.[8,10]

Processed meats, such as bacon, sausage, hot dogs, salami, luncheon meats, and liverwurst, are high in fat. They also contain sodium nitrites and salt. To check the fat content of these foods, read the label. If the food supplies more than three grams of fat for every 100 calories, it is high in fat. For example, if two turkey hot dogs provide 180 calories and eight grams of fat they are too high in fat.

Most of the fat in chicken is in the skin. The skin should be removed *before* preparation. White

| Table 13 | How To Reduce Dietary Fat | |
| --- | --- | --- |
| | **Rather Than** | **Choose To** |
| | Frying, sauteing, or cooking with oil | Bake, broil, boil, steam |
| | Making soup from homemade stock | Refrigerate stock and skim fat |
| | Basting with oil | Baste with fat-free stock, mustard, wine |
| | Using oil, butter, margarine in cooking | Saute foods in defatted chicken stock, use no-stick pans or PAM |
| | Using butter or margarine on toast | Use low-calorie jam |
| | Making sauces with cream, butter, oil, or other fats | Use nonfat milk thickened with nonfat dry milk solids or flour |
| | Using sour cream for dips | Use low-fat yogurt with lemon |
| | Selecting 4% cottage cheese | Select low-fat cottage cheese |
| | Making marinades with oil | Make marinades from lemon, tomato juice, fruit juice, soy sauce, cooking wine, or spices |
| | Using bacon, sausage, or luncheon meats | Use skinless poultry, veal, fish, dried beans, and peas |
| | Using tuna packed in oil | Use tuna canned in water |
| | Snacking on peanuts, potato chips, or other fatty snack foods | Snack on fresh fruit, vegetables, unbuttered popcorn |

*(Continued on next page)*

| Table 13 | How to Reduce Dietary Fat *(Cont.)* | |
|---|---|---|
| | **Rather Than** | **Choose To** |
| | Selecting french fries | Select baked potato with chives |
| | Selecting granola | Select shredded wheat, GrapeNuts, oatmeal, NutriGrain |
| | Grilling sandwiches in oil | Use non-stick pan or PAM |
| | Selecting ice cream | Select ice milk or sherbet |
| | Selecting doughnuts, croissants, breakfast rolls | Select bagels, low-fat bran muffins, whole wheat bread |

meat is lower in fat than dark meat, but the fat content is low in both.

Many types of fish are low in fat including bass, cod, flounder, haddock, halibut, pollock, sole, and tuna canned in water. Shellfish such as clams, oysters, crab, lobster, and scallops are also low in fat. Fattier fish include anchovies, herring, mackerel, salmon, and sardines. These fish have the same amount of fat found in red meats.

Although the link between cholesterol and cancer is not well established, it is recommended that people consume no more than 300 mg of cholesterol daily or about three to four eggs a week.[9] The yolk contains the cholesterol while the white is choleterol-free. To replace whole eggs in recipes, substitute two egg whites for each whole egg.

Meat is only one good source of protein. Other sources of protein include dried beans and peas, lentils, and soybeans. These alternatives also provide fiber and little or no fat. When combined with whole grain breads and cereals their protein content is comparable to meat.

4. Vegetable oils, butter, shortening, and other fats should be used sparingly. In cooking, bake, steam, or broil foods. Do not saute or fry foods in oils. If foods must be sauteed, saute in defatted chicken stock, wine, or water. Avoid sauces and gravies that contain fat. When making soup, place the stock in the refrigerator overnight and skim the fat from the surface in the morning. Limit the daily intake of oils and spreads to less than one pat of margarine or butter for each serving of bread. Use salad dressing sparingly or try reduced-fat varieties.

The best method for weight control, besides exercise, is to eat less fat and fatty foods. Fat supplies more than twice the calories of protein or starch. When fat is reduced in the diet, the quantity of food remains the same but the calories decrease. For example, a four ounce serving of chicken without the skin contains 100 calories less than the same amount of chicken with the skin.[108] A person can eat more food and lose weight if low-fat foods replace fattier selections. The maintenance of normal body weight is associated with a reduced risk for developing cancer.[8]

## How To Increase The Fiber In The Diet

A high fiber diet reduces the risk for developing cancer.[8,10] The best dietary sources of fiber are whole grain breads and cereals, dried beans and peas, fresh fruits and vegetables, and nuts and seeds. Each of the different fibers found in these foods, from the bran in whole wheat to the pectin in apples, contributes to health and the prevention of disease. (Table 14, page 50)

The recommendations for reducing fat in the diet will increase fiber intake. If three-quarters of the diet is foods from plant sources, and the majority of those foods come from unrefined, unprocessed sources, then the intake of fiber should be adequate. Not all the grains in the diet have to be whole grains, such as whole wheat, brown rice, and oatmeal, and not every fruit or vegetable must be high in fiber. Refined grains, such as white bread and rice, are low in fat and supply some vitamins. However, at least half of the grains in the diet should be from the whole grain varieties to guarantee adequate fiber intake.

Recommendations for fiber intake have not been established. Excessive consumption of fiber might reduce the absorption of some minerals and irritate the intestinal tract. The estimated safe and adequate amount of fiber that can be consumed daily is between 35 grams and 45 grams.[109] This amount can be obtained from the following:

| Table 14 | Fiber in Foods | | | |
|---|---|---|---|---|
| | **2 grams** | **4 grams** | **6 grams** | **8 grams** |
| **Fruits** | 1/2 cup most fruits | 1 large apple<br>1 large banana<br>1 large dried fig<br>1 cup straw-berries | | 1 cup black-berries<br>1 cup rasp-berries |
| **Vegetables** | 1/2 cup most vegetables (cooked)<br>1 cup vege-tables, raw | 1/2 cup broccoli<br>1 cup Brussels sprouts<br>1/2 cup carrots, cooked<br>1/2 cup greens, cooked<br>1 potato (medium)<br>1/2 sweet potato (medium)<br>1/2 cup winter squash | 1 ear corn | 1/2 cup green peas<br>1 large yam |
| **Breads** | 1 bran muffin<br>2 sl. whole wheat bread<br>2 cups popcorn<br>1 corn tortilla | 1 (2-1/4'') sq. cornbread | 2 slices seven grain bread | |
| **Cereals** | 1 Shred. Wheat biscuit<br>3/4 cup Corn Flakes | 2 Tbsp. Bran (unprocessed)<br>1/4 cup Grapenuts | 3/4 cup Bran Chex | 1/3 cup bran<br>1 cup Oatmeal (cooked) |
| **Pasta** | | | 1 cup pasta (whole wheat)<br>1 cup brown rice (cooked) | |
| **Beans** | 1 Tbsp nuts or seeds<br>1 rounded Tbsp peanut butter | 1/2 cup Lentils (cooked) | | 1/2 cup Beans (cooked) (pinto, kidney, etc.) |

- 6 servings of whole grain breads, cereals, and pasta (1 serving = 1 slice of bread, 1/2 cup cooked cereal or pasta, or 1 cup whole grain cold cereal) .................... 13 grams of fiber
- 4 servings of fresh fruits and vegetables (1 serving = 1 piece of fruit or vegetable, 1 cup raw, or 1/2 cup cooked) ............. 15-23 grams of fiber
- 1 serving of dried beans or peas (1 serving = 1/2 cup cooked) ................ 9 grams of fiber
  Total .................... 37-45 grams of fiber

## How To Increase Foods High In Vitamin A And Vitamin C In The Diet

Vitamin A and vitamin C might protect the body against several types of cancer and frequent consumption of foods high in these vitamins is recommended.

Vitamin A comes in two major forms. Retinol is the vitamin A in foods of animal origin such as liver. It is also found in some supplements. The carotenes, of which beta carotene is the most common, are found in fruits and vegetables. Both forms of vitamin A protect against cancer. The vitamin A content often varies depending on the color of the fruit or vegetable; a dark orange carrot has more vitamin A than a pale orange carrot. The vitamin A content of romaine lettuce is four times that of iceberg lettuce.

The vitamin C content of foods is easily destroyed. To protect the vitamin, store foods at temperatures below 40 degrees, cook in a minimal amount of water, use cooking water to make gravies or soups, do not leave food out in the air or under heat lamps, and purchase only enough food that can be consumed within a few days.

Many of the foods that are high in vitamin A are also high in vitamin C. To increase the daily intake of both vitamins:

- add a salad to the daily menu;
- drink vegetable and fruit juices;
- substitute sweet potato for white potato;
- top cereal with fresh fruit;
- select snacks of raw vegetables and fruits;
- use tomato sauce rather than white sauce on pasta;
- add chopped green pepper to chicken and tuna salads;
- serve fruit for dessert;
- include at least one dark green leafy vegetable in the daily menu.

## How To Increase The Intake Of Cruciferous Vegetables

The cruciferous vegetables, including cabbage, broccoli, and cauliflower, contain more than just fiber, and vitamin A and vitamin C. Cruciferous vegetables contain other cancer-fighting substances called indoles. Include several servings of these vegetables in the weekly menu.

## How To Avoid Salt-Cured And Smoked Foods, And Foods That Might Cause Cancer

No diet is completely free of cancer-promoting substances. It is possible, however, to minimize these substances while increasing the nutrients that protect against cancer, such as fiber, vitamin A, and vitamin C.

The consumption of salt-cured and nitrite-containing foods should be limited. These foods include processed meats, bacon, sausage, and luncheon meats.

Avoid cooking methods that promote the formation of cancer-causing substances. Charcoal broiling creates compounds believed to be carcinogenic. Broil, barbecue, and charbroil foods in moderation. When these methods for cooking are used, reduce the amount of meat to be cooked, select lean cuts of meat, cover the grill with aluminum foil and punch holes between the grids to let fat drip out. In addition, trim excess fat from meats, remove all charred portions of meat, do not overcook meats, baste foods with nonfat sauces, and use liquid smoke to flavor sauces rather than fat drippings, butter, or oil.[110]

Avoid or limit foods that might contain cancer-causing substances. Moldy foods should be discarded. Examine nuts in their shell for freshness before eating; old peanuts and other nuts might contain aflatoxin, a potent carcinogen. Some non-nutritive sweeteners, such as saccharin, might increase the risk for developing cancer. These sweeteners should be used in moderation or avoided.

Alcohol consumption is linked to cancer of the mouth, esophagus, pharynx, larynx, and liver.[32] It also causes birth defects in babies of mothers who drink. Alcohol increases the risk for cancer in those people who smoke.[111] If alcohol is included in the diet, it should be consumed in moderation.

## The Anti-Cancer Diet

A diet that is high in unrefined foods from plant sources and contains moderate amounts of low-fat foods of animal origin is an important step in a person's defense against cancer. A high-fiber, low-fat diet will provide ample amounts of the nutrients that fight cancer, such as vitamin A and vitamin C, as well as other nutrients, such as vitamin D, vitamin E, folic acid, vitamin $B_6$, iron, selenium, and zinc. This diet has only minimal amounts of the dietary components that encourage cancer. A reduction in fat is a good way to reduce unnecessary calories and maintain a healthy weight.

The individual can control several of the factors that cause cancer. Many of these factors also reduce a person's risk for developing other degenerative disorders and improve overall fitness and health.

# Notes

# Notes

# Notes

# Notes

# References

1. *Cancer Facts and Figures,* 1984. 90 Park Avenue, New York, NY 10016, American Cancer Society.
2. Wynder E, Gori G: Contribution of the environment to cancer incidence: An epidemiologic exercise. *Natl Canc Inst* 1977; 58:825-832.
3. Reddy B, Cohen L, McCoy G, et al: Nutrition and its relationship to cancer. *Adv Cancer Res* 1980; 32:237-345.
4. *Healthy People: The Surgeon General's Report on Health Promotion and Disease Prevention.* Washington DC, U.S. Department of Health, Education, and Welfare/Public Health Service, 1979, Publ. No. 79-55071, pp 60-67.
5. Garrison R, Somer E: *The Nutrition Desk Reference.* New Canaan, Conn, Keats Publishing Co, 1985, pp 127-137.
6. Walford R: The immunologic theory of aging: Current status. *Fed Proc* 1974; 33:20-20.
7. Doll R, Peto R: The causes of cancer: quantitive estimates of avoidable risks of cancer in the United States today. *J Natl Cancer Inst* 1981; 66:1192
8. *National Research Council: Diet, Nutrition, and Cancer.* 2101 Constitution Ave, NW Washington DC 20418, National Academy Press, 1982.
9. *Dietary Goals for the United States* ed 2. Select Committee on Nutrition and Human Needs, United States Senate. Washington DC, US Government Printing Office, 1977, Publ No. 052-070-04376-8.
10. American Cancer Society Special Report: *Nutrition and Cancer: Cause and Prevention.* 90 Park Avenue, New York, NY 10016, American Cancer Society Inc, February 10, 1984.
11. Willett W, MacMahon B: Diet and cancer — an overview. *N Eng J Med* 1984; 310:697-703.
12. Snowdon D, Phillips R, Warren C: Diet, obesity, and risk of fatal prostate cancer. *Am J Epidem* 1984; 120:244-250.
13. Hirayama T: Diet and cancer. *Nutr Canc* 1979; 1:67-81.

14. Finegold S, Attebery H, Sutter V: Effect of diet on human fecal flora: Comparison of Japanese and American Diets. *A J Clin Nutr* 1974; 27:1456.

15. Aries V, Crowther J, Drasar B, et al: Bacteria and etiology of cancer of the large bowel. *Gut* 1969; 10:334-335.

16. Reddy B: Dietary fat and its relationship to large bowel cancer. *Canc Res* 1981; 41:3700-3705.

17. Willett W, MacMahon B: Diet and Cancer — An overview. *N Eng J Med* 1984; 310:633-638.

18. Reddy B: Diet and excretion of bile acids. *Cancer Res* 1981; 41:3766.

19. Garrison R, Somer E: *The Nutrition Desk Reference,* New Canaan, Conn, Keats Publishing Co, 1985, p 130.

20. Phillips R: Role of lifestyle and dietary habits in risk of cancer among Seventh Day Adventists. *Cancer Res* 1975; 35:2313-2322.

21. Newell G, Ellison N (eds): *Nutrition and Cancer: Etiology and Treatment.* New York, Raven Press, 1981, pp 93-110.

22. Armstrong B, Brown J, Clarke H, et al: Diet and reproductive hormones: A study of vegetarian and nonvegetarian postmenopausal women. *JNCI* 1981; 67:761-767.

23. Cramer D, Welch W, Hutchison G, et al: Dietary animal fat in relation to ovarian cancer risk. *Obstet Gyn* 1984; 63:833-838.

24. Snowden D: Diet and ovarian cancer. *JAMA* 1985; 254:356.

25. Garrison R, Somer E: *The Nutrition Desk Reference.* New Canaan, Conn, Keats Publishing Co, 1985, pp 130-133.

26. Manousos O, Day N, Trichopoulos D, et al: Diet and colorectal cancer: A case control study in Greece. *Int J Cancer* 1983; 32:1.

27. Garrison R, Somer E: *The Nutrition Desk Reference.* New Canaan, Conn, Keats Publishing Co, 1985, pp 168-169.

28. McGill H, Geer J, Strong J: The natural history of atherosclerosis, in Kummerow F (ed) *Metabolism of*

*Lipids as Related to Atherosclerosis.* Springfield, IL, Charles C Thomas, 1965, p 36.

29. Hsu C, Kummerow F: Influence of elaidate and erucate on heart mitochondria. *Lipids* 1977; 12:486.

30. A cooperative trial in the primary prevention of ischemic heart disease using clofibrate: Report from the committee of Principal Investigators. *Br Heart J* 1978; 40:1069

31. Hinds M, Kilonel L, Hankin J, et al: Dietary cholesterol and lung cancer risk in a multiethnic population in Hawaii. *Int J Canc* 1983; 32:727-732.

32. Ames B: Dietary carcinogens and anticarcinogens. *Science* 1983; 221:1256-1262.

33. Medeloff A: Dietary fiber and health, in *Nutrition in Disease-Fiber.* Columbus, Ohio, Ross Laboratories, 1978, pp 5-15.

34. Jensen O: Colon cancer epidemiology, in Atrup and Williams (eds) *Experimental Colon Carcinogenesis.* Boca Raton, FL, CRC Press, 1983, pp 3-23.

35. Burkitt D: Fiber in the etiology of colorectal cancer, in Winawer, Schottenfeld, Sherlock (eds): *Colorectal Cancer:Prevention Epidemiology and Screening.* New York, Raven Press, 1980, pp 13-18.

36. Haenszel W, Berg J, Segi M, et al: Large bowel cancer in Hawaiian Japanese. *J Natl Canc Inst* 1973; 51:1765-1799.

37. Correa P, Haenszel W: The epidemiology of large bowel cancer. *Adv Cancer Res* 1978; 26:1-141.

38. Staszewski J, Mc Call M, Stenhouse N: Cancer mortality in 1962-1966 among Polish migrants to Australia. *Br J Canc* 1971; 25:599-618.

39. Goldin B, Adlercreutz H, Gorbach S, et al: Estrogen excretion patterns and plasma levels in vegetarian and omnivorous women. *N Eng J Med* 1982; 307:1542-1547.

40. Eastwood M, Kay R: An hypothesis for the action of dietary fiber along the gastrointestinal tract. *Am J Clin Nutr* 1979; 32:364-367.

41. Thomsen L, Roberton A, Wong J, et al: Intra-caecal short chain fatty acids are altered by dietary pectin in the rat. *Digestion* 1984; 29:129-137.

42. Bjelke E: Dietary vitamin A and human lung cancer. *Int J Cancer* 1975; 15:561.

43. Graham S, Marshall J, Mettlin C, et al: Diet in the epidemiology of breast cancer. *Am J Epidemiol* 1982; 116:68.

44. Garrison R, Somer E: *The Nutrition Desk Reference*. New Canaan, Conn, Keats Publishing Co, 1985, pp 139-140.

45. Basu T: Vitamin A and cancer of epithelial origin. *J Human Nutr* 1979; 33:24-31.

46. Weber F: Biochemical mechanisms of vitamin A action. *Proc Nutr Soc* 1983; 42:31-41.

47. Basu T, Chan U, Fields A: Vitamin A (retinol) and epithelial cancer in man, in Prasad (ed): *Vitamins, Nutrition, and Cancer.* Basel, Switzerland, Karger Publishers, 1984, pp 33-45.

48. Kummet T, Meyskens F: Vitamin A: A potential inhibitor of human cancer. *Seminars in Oncology* 1983; 10:281.

49. Shekelle R, Liu S, Raynor W, et al: Dietary vitamin A and risk of cancer in the Western Electric Study. *Lancet* 1981; 2:1185-1189.

50. Dungal N, Sigurjonsson J: Gastric cancer and diet: A pilot study on dietary habits in two districts differing markedly in respect of mortality from gastric cancer. *Br J Cancer* 1967; 21:270.

51. Hormozdiari H, Day N, Aramesh B, et al: Dietary factors and esophageal cancer in the Caspian Littoral of Iran. *Cancer Res* 1975; 35:3493.

52. Tuyns A: Protective effect of citrus fruit on esophageal cancer. *Nutr Cancer* 1983; 5:195-200.

53. Yamanaka W: Vitamin C and Cancer: How convincing a connection? *Postgrad Med* 1985; 78:47-53.

54. Committee on Nitrite and Alternative Curing Agents in Foods, National Academy of Science-National Research Council: *The Health Effects of Nitrate, Nitrite and N-Nitroso Compounds,* Washington DC, National Academy Press, 1981.

55. Cameron E, Pauling L, Leibovitz B: Ascorbic acid and cancer: A review. *Cancer Res* 1979; 39:663-681.

56. Schlegel J: Proposed uses of ascorbic acid in the prevention of bladder carcinoma. *Ann NY Acad Sci* 1975; 258:432-437.

57. Dion P: The effect of dietary ascorbic acid and alpha-tocopherol on fecal mutagenicity. *Mutat Res* 1982; 102:27-37.

58. Howatson A, Carter D: High fat, protein-diet and pancreatic carcinogenesis. *Gut* 1983; 24:A985.

59. Cunningham A: Lymphomas and animal protein consumption. *Lancet* 1976; 2:1184.

60. Czajka-Nfarins D, Cheney C, Aker S: Nutrition, diet and cancer, in Krause M, Mahan L (eds): *Food, Nutrition, and Diet Therapy* 7 ed. Philadelphia, WB Saunders, 1984, pp 735-743.

61. Merz B: Adding seeds to the diet may keep cancer at bay. *JAMA* 1983; 249:2746.

62. Shamberger R: Vitamins and Cancer: Current controversies. *The Cancer Bulletin* 1982; 34:150-154.

63. Garland C, Shekelle R, Barrett-Connor E, et al: Dietary vitamin D and calcium and risk of colorectal cancer: A 19 year prospective study in men. *Lancet* 1985; 1:307-309.

64. Prasad D, Edwards-Prasad J: Effects of tocopherol (vitamin E) acid succinate or morphological alterations and growth inhibition in melanoma cells in culture. *Canc Res* 1983; 42:550-555.

65. Horvath P, Clement L: Synergistic effect of vitamin E and selenium in the chemoprevention of mammary carcinogenesis in rats. *Canc Res* 1983; 43:5335-5541.

66. Garrison R, Somer E: *The Nutrition Desk Reference.* New Canaan, Conn, Keats Publishing Co, 1985, pp 40-42.

67. Yunis J, Soreng A: Constitutive fragile sites in cancer. *Science* 1984; 226:1199-1204.

68. Butterworth C: Folate-induced regression of cervical intraepithelial neoplasias in users of oral contraceptive agents. *Am J Clin Nutr* 1980; 32:926.

69. Tamura T, Stokstad E: Folic acid. *Nutrition and the MD* 1984; 10:13.

70. Hendler S: *The Complete Guide to Anti-aging Nutrients.* New York, Simon and Schuster, 1985, pp 99-100.

71. Prior F: Theoretical involvement of vitamin B6 in tumor initiation. *Medical Hypothesis.* 1985; 16:421-428.

72. Briggs G, Calloway D: *Nutrition and Physical Fitness* ed 10. Philadelphia, WB Saunders Company, 1973, p 194.

73. Pao E, Mickle S: Problem nutrients in the United States. *Food Tech* 1981; Sept.

74. *Nationwide Food Consumption Survey,* Spring 1980. Beltsville, MD, US Dept Agriculture, Science and Education Administration.

75. Garrison R, Somer E: *The Nutrition Desk Reference.* New Canaan, Conn, Keats Publishing Co, 1985, pp 66-68, 116-123.

76. The National Research Council, Committee on Dietary Allowances, Food and Nutrition Board: *Recommended Dietary Allowances* ed 9. Washington DC, National Academy of Sciences, 1980, pp 137-144.

77. Schrauzer G, Ishmael D: Effects of selenium and of arsenic on the genesis of spontaneous mammary tumors in inbred C3H mice. *Ann Clin Lab Sci* 1974; 4:441.

78. Shamberger R, Tytko S, Willis C: Antioxidants and cancer: VI Selenium and age-adjusted human cancer mortality. *Arch Environ Health* 1976; 31:231.

79. Schrauzer G, White D, Schneider C: Cancer mortality correlation studies. III: Statistical associates with dietary selenium intakes. *Bioniorg Chem* 1977; 7:23-24.

80. Shamberger R, Rukovena E, Longfield A, et al: Antioxidants and cancer: I. Selenium in the blood of normals and cancer patients. *JNCI* 1973; 50:863.

81. Garrison R, Somer E: *The Nutrition Desk Reference.* New Canaan, Conn, Keats Publishing Co, 1985, pp 140-141.

82. Willett W, Polk B, Harris J, et al: Prediagnostic serum selenium and risk of cancer. *Lancet* 1983; 2:130-134.

83. Griffin A: Role of selenium in the chemoprevention of cancer. *Adv Canc Res* 1979; 29:419-442.

84. Spalholz J: Selenium: What role in immunity and immune cytotoxicity, in Spalholz J, Martin J, Ganther H (eds): *Selenium in Biology and Medicine.* Westport, Conn, AVI Publishing, 1981, pp 103-117.

85. Helzlsouer K: Selenium and cancer prevention. *Seminars in Oncology* 1983; 10:308.

86. Noda M, Takano T, Sakurai H: Effects of selenium on chemical carcinogens. *Mut Res* 1979:66:175.

87. Garrison R, Somer E: *The Nutrition Desk Reference.* New Canaan, Conn, Keats Publishing Co, 1985, pp 77-78.

88. Allen J, Bell E, Oken M, et al: Zinc deficiency, hyperzincuria and immune dysfunction in lung cancer patients. *Am J Clin Nutr* 1983; 37:720.

89. Oleske J: Plasma zinc and copper in primary and secondary immunodeficiency disorders. *Biol Tr El Res* 1983; l5:189-194.

90. Whelan P, Walker B, Kelleher J: Zinc, vitamin A, and prostatic cancer. *Br J Urol* 1983; 55:525-528.

91. Chandra R: Excessive intake of zinc impairs immune responses. *JAMA* 1984; 252:1443-1446.

92. Hamilton S, Hyland J, McAvinchey D, et al: Effects of dietary beer or ethanol on experimental colonic carcinogenesis. *Gastroentry* 1983; 84:1180.

93. Hausman P: *Foods That Fight Cancer.* New York, Rawson Associates, 1983, pp 121-133.

94. Garrison R, Somer E: *The Nutrition Desk Reference.* New Canaan, Conn, Keats Publishing Co, 1985, pp 135-137.

95. Talamini R, LaVecchia C, Decarli A, et al: Social factors, diet and breast cancer in a northern Italian population. *Br J Cancer* 1984; 49:723-729.

96. Alexander L, Goff H: Chemicals, cancer, and cytochrome P-450. *J Chem Ed* 1982; 59:179.

97. Garrison R, Somer E: *The Nutrition Desk Reference.* New Canaan, Conn., Keats Publishing Co., 1985, p 210.

98. Weisburger J, Wynder E, Horn C: Nutrition and Cancer — A review of relevant mechanisms. *Canc Bul* 1982; 34:128-136.

99. Bristol J, Emmett P, Heaton K, et al: Sugar, fat, and the risk of colorectal cancer. *Br Med J* 1985; 291:1467-1470.

100. Sugary foods may promote breast cancer. *New Scientist,* March 10, 1983, p 648.

101. Doyle R, Redding J: *The Complete Food Handbook.* New York, Grove Press, 1976, pp 237, 326.

102. Concon J, Newburg D, Swerczek T: Black Pepper (Piper Nigrum) Evidence of Carcinogenicity. *Nutr Cancer* 1979; 1:22.

103. Levin D, Hollstein M, Christman M, et al: A new salmonella tester strain (TA102) with A-T base parts at the site of mutagen detects oxidative mutagens. *Proc Natl Acad Sci USA.* 1982; 79:7445.

104. Jadhav S, Sharma R, Salunkhe K: Naturally occuring toxic alkaloids in foods. *CRC Crit Rev Toxicol* 1981; 9:212.

105. Lin R, Kessler I: A multifactorial model for pancreatic cancer in man: Epidemiologic evidence. *JAMA* 1981; 245:147.

106. MacMahon B: Coffee and cancer of the pancreas. *N Eng J Med* 1981; 304:630.

107. Jacobsen B, Bjelke E: Coffee consumption and cancer: A prospective study. Presented at the 13th International Cancer Congress, Seattle, 1982.

108. *Nutritive Value of American Foods: In Common Units.* Agriculture Handbook No. 456. Washington DC, US Department of Agriculture, 1975, Publ. No. 001-000-03184.

109. Garrison R, Somer E: *The Nutrition Desk Reference.* New Canaan, Conn, Keats Publishing Co, 1985, pp 189-190.

110. *Facts You Should Know About: Outdoor Cooking.* Washington DC, American Institute for Cancer Research, 1985.

111. *Healthy People: The Surgeon General's Report on Health Promotion and Disease Prevention.* Washington DC, US Department of Health, Education, and Welfare/Public Health Service. 1979, Publication No. 79-55071, p 62.

112. Ibid, p viii.

113. *Chemical Cuisine.* 1755 S. St., NW, Washington, DC 20009, Center For Science In The Public Interest.

# Glossary

**Aflatoxin:** A mold that is carcinogenic and is found in stale nuts and other stale foods.

**Antioxidant:** A compound, such as selenium, vitamin E, or vitamin C, that protects other compounds or tissues from the destructive effects of oxygen derivatives.

**Benzo{a}pyrene:** A carcinogen formed when foods are broiled or are cooked at high temperatures over a grill.

**Beta carotene:** The form of vitamin A found in foods from plant sources such as carrots and dark green leafy vegetables.

**Cancer:** The uncontrolled growth of abnormal cells.

**Carcinogen:** A substance that causes cancer.

**Cardiovascular disease:** A disease of the heart and blood vessels caused by the accumulation of cholesterol in the lining of the blood vessels.

**Cellulose:** A type of fiber in foods from plant sources.

**Cholesterol:** A type of fat found in foods from animal sources and produced by the body. High levels of cholesterol in the blood are associated with the development of cardiovascular disease.

**Cruciferous:** A vegetable that belongs to the cabbage family, including broccoli, asparagus, cauliflower, and cabbage.

**Cyclamates:** Non-nutritive sweeteners that are carcinogenic and banned from use in foods.

**Diabetes:** A disorder in which the body's ability to use sugar is impaired because of inadequate production or utilization of the hormone insulin.

**Epithelial:** The internal and external surfaces of the body, including the skin, lining of the blood vessels, and outer surface of the eyes.

**Esophagus:** The passageway from the throat to the stomach.

**Estrogen:** A female sex hormone that helps regulate ovulation and sex characteristics.

**Free Radical:** A highly reactive compound derived from air pollution, radiation, cigarette smoke, or the incomplete breakdown of proteins and fats; reacts with fats in cell membranes and changes their shape and function.

**Guar gum:** A type of fiber in foods from plant sources.

**Hemicellulose:** A type of fiber in foods from plant sources.

**Hormone:** A chemical substance produced by a group of cells or an organ called an endocrine gland, that is released into the blood and transported to another organ or tissue, where it performs a specific action. Examples are insulin, estrogen, adrenalin.

**Hydrogenated Fat:** An unsaturated vegetable fat that has been processed to become more saturated, such as margarine and shortening.

**Hypertension:** High blood pressure.

**Immune system:** A complex system of substances, such as antibodies, white blood cells, and lymphocytes, and tissues that protect the body from disease and infection.

**Lignin:** A type of fiber in foods from plant sources.

**Lymph system:** A system of lymph vessels, fluid, and nodes that removes debris and cellular waste products from the blood and cells. The filtered lymph fluid is returned to the blood.

**Metastasis:** The spread of disease (cancer) from one location in the body to another.

**Nitrite:** A compound found naturally in some foods or added as a preservative and coloring agent to processed meats. A nitrite is converted in the stomach to the carcinogen nitrosamine.

**Nitrosamines:** Substances that cause cancer and are found naturally in the environment or produced from dietary nitrites in the stomach.

**Oxidation:** A chemical process where a substance combines with oxygen.

**Pectin:** A type of fiber in foods from plant sources.

**Polyunsaturated fat:** A type of unsaturated fat.

**Prostate:** An organ surrounding the neck of the bladder and the beginning of the urethra in the male. This gland secretes a fluid that nourishes and hastens the movement of semen through the urethra.

**Saturated Fat:** A type of fat that is solid at room temperature and is found in foods from animal sources, hydrogenated vegetable oils, and coconut or palm oil. A diet high in these fats is linked to the development of cardiovascular disease and cancer.

**Tocopherol:** Vitamin E.

**Unsaturated Fat:** A type of fat that is liquid at room temperature and is found in foods from plant sources such as vegetable oils, nuts, and seeds.

# Index

## A

Aflatoxin, p 5, 38, 53
Air Pollution, p 13
Alcohol, p 4, 5, 8, 41,
33, 53
   and vitamin A, p 34
   and vitamin C, p 34
   and B vitamins, p 34
   and selenium, p 34
   and zinc, p 34
Animal Fat, p 25
Antioxidants, p 17, 22,
31
Aspartame, p 35, 36

## B

B Vitamins, p 34
(See Specific B Vitamin)
Benzo(a)pyrenes, p 5, 39
Beta Carotene, p 5, 18,
19, 21, 51
   and cell membranes, p
20
   sources, p 18, 19
Bile, p 10, 17
Bladder Cancer:
   and beta carotene, p 18
   and caffeine, p 38
   and selenium, p 31
   and sweeteners, p 35
   and vitamin A, p 20
   and vitamin C, p 22
Breast Cancer:
   and alcohol, p 33
   and beta carotene, p 18
   and body weight, p 8
   and fat, p 9, 11, 12,
     15, 16
   and fiber, p 15, 16
   and estrogen, p 15
   and selenium, p 30, 31
   and sugar, p 35
   and vegetable protein,
     p 24
   and vegetarians, p 15
   and vitamin A, p 20
   and vitmain D, p 25

## C

Cadmium, p 31
Caffeine, p 38
Cardiovascular Disease, p
7
   and fat, p 42
   and fiber, p 42
   and polyunsaturated
     fats, p 13
Cell Membranes, p 13,
19, 26
Cellulose, p 16, 17, 50
Cervical Cancer, p 8
   and beta carotene, p 18
   and body weight, p 8
   and vitamin A, p 20
Cholesterol, p 10, 13, 15,
     44, 45, 47,
   sources, p 14
Cigarette Smoking, p 4,
39
   and alcohol, p 33, 53
   and beta carotene, p 20
   and nitrosamines, p 35
   and vitamin C, p 21

Colon Cancer, p 10, 13, 35
  and alcohol, p 33, 53
  and animal protein, p 24, 25
  and body weight, p 8
  and cholesterol, p 13
  and fat, p 9, 10, 15, 16
  and fiber, p 15, 16
  and selenium, p 31
  and vegetable protein, p 24
  and vegetarians, p 19
  and vitamin A, p 20
  and vitamin C, p 22
  and vitamin D, p 25
Cruciferous Vegetables, p 8, 22, 23, 41, 52
Cytochrome, P-450, p 33

**D**

Diabetes, p 7, 42

**E**

Epithelial Tissues, p 20
Esophageal Cancer:
  and alcohol, p 33, 53
  and beta carotene, p 18
  and nitrosamines, p 34
Estrogen, p 26

**F**

Fat, p 4, 5, 8, 11, 12, 15, 16, 18, 23, 25, 26, 35, 38, 39, 41, 42-47, 48, 53, 54,
  cholesterol, p 10

sources, p 9, 10
Fatty Acids, p 16, 17
Fiber, p 4, 5, 8, 9, 11, 12, 15, 16, 18, 21, 23, 25, 35, 41, 42, 43, 44, 49-53
  cellulose, p 16, 17, 50
  hemicellulose, p 16, 17
  lignin, p 16, 17
  pectin, p 16, 17, 50
  gums, p 16, 17
  estrogen, p 15
  sources, p 49, 50, 51
Folic Acid, p 23, 27, 54
  sources, p 27, 29
Food Additives, p 36
Free Radicals, p 13
  and lignin, p 17
  and polyunsaturated fats, p 13
  and selenium, p 31
  and vitamin C, p 32
  and vitamin E, p 25, 26

**G**

Gall Bladder Cancer, p 8
Geniteal Tract Cancer, p 31
Gums (fiber), p 16, 17

**H**

Heart Disease (See Cardiovascular Disease)
Hemicellulose, p 16, 17
Hodgkins Disease, p 31
Hypertension, p 42

# I

Immune System, p 4, 40
  and alcohol, p 34
  and beta carotene, p 19
  and iron, p 30
  and selenium, p 31
  and vitamin $B_6$, p 27
  and vitamin C, p 22
  and zinc, p 32
Indoles, p 22, 23
Iron, p 23, 54

# K

Kidney Cancer, p 8

# L

Larynx Cancer:
  and alcohol, p 33, 53
  and beta carotene, p 18
  and vitamin A, p 20
Lignin, p 16, 17
Liver Cancer:
  and aflatoxin, p 38
  and alcohol, p 53
  and vegetable protein,
    p 24
Lung Cancer:
  and beta carotene, p
    18, 20
  and selenium, p 30
  and vitamin A, p 20
  and zinc, p 32
Lymphoma:
  and selenium, p 30, 31
  and vegetable progein,
    p 25

# M

Metals, p 5
  and selenium, p 31
Mercury, p 31
Metastasis, p 1, 2
Mouth Cancer:
  and alcohol, p 33, 53
  and beta carotene, p 18
  and vitamin A, p 20

# N

Natural Carcinogens, p
  37, 38
Nitrosamines, p 4, 5, 34
  nitrates, p 5, 8, 34, 41,
    45, 52
  nitrites, p 5, 34
  and vitamin C, p 21,
    35
  and vitamin E, p 35

# O

Obesity, p 18, 42
Ovarian Cancer, p 9, 12
Oxidation, p 13, 22

# P

Pancreatic Cancer:
  and animal protein, p
    24
  and caffeine, p 38
Pectin, p 16, 17
Pesticides, p 5, 37
Pharynx, p 33, 53
Piperine, p 37
Polychlorinated Biphenyl
  (PCB), p 5, 37

Polyunsaturated Fat, p 12, 13, 26
Polyvinylchloride (PVC), p 5
Processed Foods, p 8, 27
  and folic acid, p 27
  and vitamin B$_6$, p 28
Prostrate Cancer, p 8
  and animal protein, p 24
  and body weight, p 8
  and fat, p 8, 9, 12
  and vitamin A, p 20
  and zinc, p 32
Protease Inhibitors, p 24
Protein, p 13, 27, 28, 29, 47, 48
  animal, p 24, 25
  vegetable, p 23, 24, 25
Pyridoxime (See Vitamin B$_6$)

**R**

Radiation, p 13
Retinol, p 18, 51
Riboflavin (See Vitamin B$_2$)

**S**

Safrole, p 37
Salt Cured, p 8, 41, 45, 52
Saturated Fat, p 12, 13, 44, 45
Selenium, p 4, 23, 26, 30, 31, 32, 34, 54
  sources, p 31
  toxicity, p 32
Skin Cancer, p 31

Smoked Foods, p 39, 41, 52
Stomach Cancer:
  and body weight, p 8
  and iron, p 30
  and nitrosamines, p 35
  and selenium, p 31
  and vitamin A, p 20
  and vitamin C, p 21
Sugar, p 8, 42, 35
Sweeteners, p 5, 35, 36, 53

**T**

Tannic Acid, p 5
Thiamin (See Vitamin B$_1$)
Throat Cancer, p 20
Trans-Fatty Acids, p 13

**U**

Unsaturated Fat, p 12
Uterine Cancer:
  and body weight, p 8
  and fat, p 9, 12
Urinary Tract Cancer, p 35

**V**

Vegetarians, p 15, 19
Vitamin A, p 4, 5, 23, 34, 41, 43, 52, 54
(See Also Beta Carotene)
  carotenoids, p 18, 51
  and epithelial tissues, p 20
  retinol, p 18
  sources, p 21
  toxicity, p 21

Vitamin B$_6$, p 23, 27, 54
Vitamin C, p 4, 5, 23,
    34, 35, 41, 43, 52, 54
  sources, p 22, 23, 51
Vitamin D, p 23, 54
Vitamin E, p 5, 23, 25,
    26, 27, 28, 35, 54
  and cell membranes, p
    26
  and fat, p 26

and selenium, p 26
and polyunsaturated
    fat, p 26
sources, p 27, 29

## Z

Zinc, p 23, 34, 54
  sources, p 32